Food Rules for The Right Diet: The Simple Guide For A Healthy Life

How to Eat Right for A Long Life

By: Jason Craig

TABLE OF CONTENTS

Publishers Notes.. 3

Dedication 4

Chapter 1- Understanding the Dangers of Genetically
Engineered Foods 5

Chapter 2- The Most Deadly Foods and Why You Should Stay
Away From Them...13

Chapter 3- How to Improve Your Digestion.......................18

Chapter 4- Cleaning Our Kidneys with the Right Foods – Detox
Foods 22

Chapter 5- Understanding How to Use Free Radicals for Healthy
Eating Habits...25

Chapter 6- The Truth about Healthy Cholesterols 28

Chapter 7- Top Ten Tips for a Healthier You....................30

About The Author...34

Jason Craig

PUBLISHERS NOTES

Disclaimer

This publication is intended to provide helpful and informative material. It is not intended to diagnose, treat, cure, or prevent any health problem or condition, nor is intended to replace the advice of a physician. No action should be taken solely on the contents of this book. Always consult your physician or qualified health-care professional on any matters regarding your health and before adopting any suggestions in this book or drawing inferences from it.

The author and publisher specifically disclaim all responsibility for any liability, loss or risk, personal or otherwise, which is incurred as a consequence, directly or indirectly, from the use or application of any contents of this book.

Any and all product names referenced within this book are the trademarks of their respective owners. None of these owners have sponsored, authorized, endorsed, or approved this book.

Always read all information provided by the manufacturers' product labels before using their products. The author and publisher are not responsible for claims made by manufacturers.

© 2013

Manufactured in the United States of America

DEDICATION

This book is dedicated to those who want to be happy, healthy and at the right weight.

Jason Craig

Chapter 1- Understanding the Dangers of Genetically Engineered Foods

In the past two centuries, human comprehension of the universe has far outstripped society's attempts to either contain or completely assimilate it. One need look no further than Toffler's concept of "future shock" and the unrelenting controversy over the all-but-proven theory of evolution to see this in action. Our application of recently-acquired knowledge to new technologies, including atomic energy, electronics, computers, telephony, and medicine, have all greatly affected our species, often in ways that we do not yet fully understand.

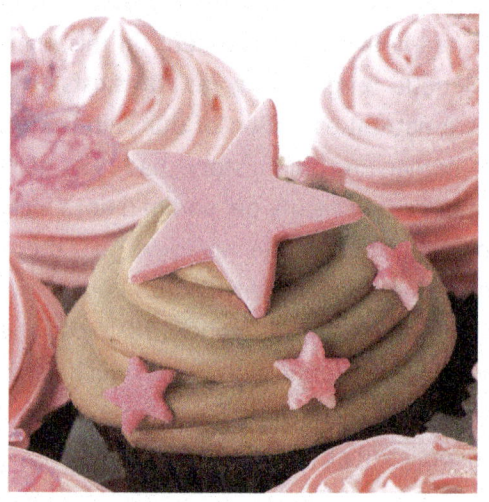

While showing signs of uniting us as a species, this rapid evolution of technology also has the potential to divide us. Few technologies better illustrate this double-edged promise than genetic engineering, the science that that has given us genetically modified or "GM" food crops. As opposed to biotechnology, which uses existing organisms and their by-products to make foods (a practice

Food Rules for The Right Diet

as old as the manufacture of wine, beer, cheese, and yogurt), genetic engineering involves actually changing an organism's genome.

While some hail GM foods as a godsend, others find them repugnant, for reasons both religious and practical. This article will briefly examine arguments from both sides of the GM foods divide. Its viewpoint is primarily environmental, though it must be pointed out that social and economic effects are not entirely ignored, since humans are a significant part of the modern environment.

Arguments for GM Foods

One of the things that make us human is our tendency to manipulate our environment to our advantage. All creatures do this to some extent, but none more so than human beings. Collectively, this is known as culture, and over time it has allowed us to conquer nearly every environment on this planet, and a few outside it. Genetic engineering as it exists today may be understood as a natural evolution of our culture, and might have begun much earlier in our history had we gained a better understanding of genetics early on, and had not elected to develop chemical and mechanical technology at the expense of biotechnology. Indeed, if Gregor Mendel's observations about pea plants hadn't been forgotten or ignored for most of a century, it's likely that by now we would have been much farther along the road toward full-fledged GM foods -- so far along, in fact, that the current controversies might be moot.

In a sense, genetically modifying our food is nothing new; humans have been doing it for more than 10,000 years, ever since we learned how to strengthen existing biological traits by breeding plants or animals that best exemplified those traits. For example, corn initially resulted from a fortuitous cross between Mexican

Jason Craig

teosinte and gamagrass, but has been extensively developed by humans since.

This type of genetic modification is a slow process of breeding the best and weeding out the failures, but it's still genetic modification, if only of the crudest sort. Modern genetic modification is much faster, and is performed using recombinant DNA techniques, which produces new DNA; apparently, it's this that most frightens the opponents of GM foods. It's human nature to be frightened of the unknown, but GM foods also offer many positive aspects to be embraced.

One example is the potential to make existing crops hardier, better able to handle climate change and pests in particular. Mother Nature is quite efficient at adapting existing organisms to various environments, but she doesn't work for us and tends to make her changes on a geological timescale. However, some climatic changes do occur rather quickly even on a human timescale, especially in these days when humans have a direct and observable affect on the worldwide environment; and we don't have time to wait dozens of generations for a food crop to develop a resistance to cold, drought, or blight on its own. Genetically modifying its genome allows us to make this change in just a few generations at most.

GM foods have direct benefits for human beings as well. Imagine foods with longer shelf lives, corn with a higher nutritive value, rice that stimulates our bodies to produce much-needed Vitamin A, or vegetables that produce oils naturally low in saturated fats. These are already being developed, and decidedly odd options such as "edible vaccines" (in the form of a special GM fruit, such as a banana, to which the vaccine has been genetically added) are being explored. Furthermore, since GM crops are less likely to be contaminated with toxins (they require fewer chemicals to grow), they're also safer to eat.

Food Rules for The Right Diet

GM crops can also be of great benefit to farmers -- because, as mentioned, they require fewer herbicides, pesticides, fertilizers, and fuel for their cultivation. Genes to resist freezing, drought, and pests can significantly increase crop yields, certainly an important factor in a world teeming with nearly seven billion people. Even 5-8 percent greater yields, which have been reported for some GM crops, can translate into millions more people fed. Viewed from an economic perspective, that would equal billions more dollars per year for farmers as well.

According to proponents, cultivation of GM crops can have beneficial effects for the environment, too. They point out that if modern farmers went to more widespread use of GM crops, the amount of agricultural chemicals contaminating the environment would drop sharply, leaving our waterways, forests, and fields cleaner and fuller of life. Fewer chemicals would also benefit our oceans, which can no longer easily absorb our chemical wastes; the growing "Dead Zone" in the Gulf of Mexico is proof enough of this. The Dead Zone is characterized by a lack of dissolved oxygen and thus very little sea life, the result of chemical fertilizers carried into the Gulf by the Mississippi River.

A less obvious benefit of GM foods is the fact that if crop yields are larger, then the same amount of land can feed more people. That means it's unnecessary to clear more land for agriculture, leaving it in place for plant and animal habitat, soil conservation, recreation, and other uses. If croplands are used more efficiently because of their widespread adoption, GM plants can also decrease erosion and other environmental impacts, simply because the fields are cleared less often.

One final argument for GM foods is that they happen to be the most tightly regulated foods in the industry. In-depth analyses are required before a GM food is allowed to be sold, in order to ensure that it meets federal standards, and the process takes years. The regulatory process is extremely rigorous, particularly in the United States and Europe, so any purported environmental, health, or social impacts should be minimal.

Arguments against GM Foods

Some of the arguments against GM foods are based on the belief that splicing foreign genes into an organism is "unnatural" or "immoral." These arguments are more social than empirical, however: for example, some claim that we're intruding on the realm of the Creator when we modify an organism's genome, and others worry about how GM foods might impact dietary laws. Because these arguments so strongly affect humans, they cannot be ignored; however, there are more important reasons why raising GM foods might ultimately be a mistake.

One argument that's familiar to many Americans (if only because it was advocated by the Ian Malcolm character in the movie Jurassic Park) is that adding a GM organism to the ecosystem will almost certainly have unpredictable results. The current ecosystem is a balance of species and forces that evolved over millions of years, and adding new organisms indiscriminately could unsettle this balance. We humans already seriously impact the environment with our activities and wastes; GM organisms can be viewed just another form of pollutant. After little more than a decade of growing GM foods, we still have no good idea of their long-term environmental effects. Are GM foods really safe, either for humans or their environment?

Some GM foods could pose health risks to some people. Take, for example, peanut allergies: they can be so deadly that a few bites of peanut butter can kill an allergy sufferer. Supposed a GM food contained the peanut genes that caused the reaction? If it were improperly labeled, it might cause numerous deaths before it was pulled off the market. More significantly, the bacteria quietly living in one's body could incorporate the antibacterial genes often used in GM food as genetic markers. If this happened, new antibiotic-resistant strains of bacteria might take hold and spread. This might result in new or revitalized diseases ravaging their way through human populations, or escaping into the ecosystem and similarly impacting wild plants and animals.

Critics counter the claim that GM foods will help farmers by pointing out that they're far more likely to benefit agribusinesses than small farmers, simply because the initial outlay is extremely costly. Nor are the environmental benefits as clear as some advocates claim. For one thing, GM crops contribute to the trend toward "monoculture," in which just a few crops provide most of the world's food. Not only does this decrease biodiversity in the environment at large, it can leave much of our food supply at the mercy of a single disease or insect pest. Suppose a new form of blight, resistant to pesticides because it had evolved a natural immunity to the pesticide genes used in GM plants, raged through the world's corn or rice crops? Millions of people would die, because they count on those plants for most of their daily food intake.

GM crops also have the potential to harm the environment in other ways. One fear is the "superweeds" that might result from accidental cross-fertilization between GM crops and ordinary plants. Some species of wild plants, especially grasses, are closely related to species we grow as food crops, and can share genetic material. If a grass were to obtain an herbicide-resistant gene, it might become nearly impossible to kill, short of pulling up each and every stalk. Worse, even plants that aren't related to each other can trade genes, if viruses get into the act. Viruses work by getting into a cell and then turning into a virus factory. If a particular virus could infect two unrelated plants -- for example, corn and canola -- traits from one could be transferred to the other via viral mechanisms.

These are more than alarmist fantasies, because there are already cases of GM plants acting as "superweeds." In Canada, GM canola plants have begun invading nearby non-GM wheat fields. More to the point, what may be a true herbicide-resistant "superweed" has recently been identified in fields used to grow GM crops in England, though scientists say that there is no evidence it can produce viable seeds. In many parts of the world, including the U.S., Europe, and Asia, genes from GM corn have been found to have contaminated unmodified corn via cross-pollination.

Another worry is the effect of GM crops on animal pests, particularly insects. Bt corn, a popular GM crop developed from corn naturally resistant to the corn borer worm, also has a deleterious effect on monarch butterfly larvae, at least when the caterpillars are fed Bt corn leaves in the laboratory. This is alarming, because monarch butterflies migrate across the U.S. "Corn Belt," where Bt corn is in common use. Fortunately monarch butterflies eat milkweed leaves almost exclusively, so the effect hasn't been pronounced in the natural population.

Nonetheless, these findings raise serious issues about how these plants will affect other insects. Bt toxin does not discriminate; it might kill beneficial creatures as often as it kills pests. Alternately, it may generate some rapid cases of microevolution, in which bugs naturally resistant to the toxin survive to produce a generation of "superbugs" that can wipe a Bt cornfield clean in days.

Like most significant scientific breakthroughs, GM foods are a mixed blessing. On the one hand, they could help save humanity from itself; on the other, they may well hasten our demise, and that of most other naturally evolved organisms on this planet. But as with nuclear power, the genie is out of the bottle; all we can do now is walk the narrow path between salvation and disaster. We have proven up to the task with the nuclear genie, at least so far; let us hope we can do the same with the GM genie.

Food Rules for The Right Diet

The carrying capacity of the Earth -- that is, the number of people it can sustain using standard subsistence farming methods -- has long since been exceeded. Only the "Green Revolution" and constant development of new chemical pesticides, herbicides, and fertilizers has kept us in the game. Lacking a unified world government and a series of draconian birth-control measures, it seems unlikely that the human population will decrease significantly anytime soon, especially in developing nations where large families are traditional and, for social reasons, often necessary. Therefore, it seems that we must take our chances with GM foods for now, though this is not to say that they shouldn't be tightly regulated at all times. Given the number of mouths the world must feed, GM foods may be humanity's only hope for short-term survival, at least until we can develop new sources of food production -- whether they be more extensive aquaculture, vat-grown foods, or domed farms on the moon and under the sea.

Furthermore, GM foods may be the only way to save at least a portion of the environment unaltered for posterity. In the past few decades, humanity as a group has become much more aware of the importance of environmental health; however, our population continues to expand, even as efforts are made to slow environmental degradation. Unless we take a few chances, like the ones that come with GM foods, it may be too late to avoid permanently fouling the only nest we have.

Chapter 2- The Most Deadly Foods and Why You Should Stay Away From Them

Alzheimer's disease, cancer, attention deficit hyperactivity disorder and autism are plaguing our society. Countless diseases are ravaging our bodies and there is no definite cure in sight. Is there any hope that our society can return to a state of good health?

We, as the American people, are steadily eating ourselves to death. The foods we consume are laced with toxins that are slowly poisoning our bodies. These toxic ingredients have been approved by the Food and Drug Administration for use in the foods that we consume every day.

A common toxin found in today's foods is phenylalanine, which can cause seizures, brain damage and mental retardation in people who are sensitive to its effects or have phenylketonuria (PKU.) It is in a category of additives called excitotoxins. Excitotoxins are chemicals added to our foods to enhance flavor. These toxins cause direct harm to nerve cells, causing the cells to become over-excited to the point of death of the cells. While phenylalanine is naturally occurring in some foods, it is also an ingredient added to man-made foods, such as artificial sweetener (aspartame) used in diet soft drinks, diet foods and some medicines.

Due to the potential for health problems associated with the use of phenylalanine, products containing this ingredient are labeled with special warnings. The best course of action concerning this dangerous ingredient is to avoid it at all costs. Choose foods and drinks that do not contain aspartame or phenylalanine.

Diacetyl is another detrimental ingredient in the American diet, and also a part of the excitotoxin family of food chemicals. Diacetyl (butanedione) is used in the flavoring process of foods, such as pet foods, microwave popcorn and candies, among others. Studies have shown that many food processing plant employees, who come into contact with food flavorings containing diacetyl (FFCD) on a regular basis, suffer with serious respiratory illnesses. Some of the health issues caused by FFCD include wheezing, shortness of breath and a persistent dry cough. A high percentage of these employees developed asthma or bronchiolitis obliterans. Bronchiolitis obliterans results in inflammation and scarring of small airways, which causes the airways to become thick and narrow. This is a permanent condition which cannot be reversed.

Many of the employees working in microwave popcorn processing plants have been treated for eye, nasal, or upper respiratory irritation or burns, due to exposure to the vapors emitted by the FFCD.

Testing involving FFCD has shown respiratory tract damage and death in rodents that were exposed to diacetyl and diacetyl-laced butter flavorings. Further testing has also shown that rats that are exposed to 198.4 ppm (parts per million) of diacetyl for only six hours suffered from necrosis (localized death of living tissue) of the nasal and tracheal epithelium (membranous tissues that line the nasal and tracheal passages.)

A third member of the excitotoxin family, monosodium glutamate (MSG), can cause headaches, numbness and burning in the neck, face and other areas, heart palpitations, nausea, chest pains, and general weakness. MSG is commonly found in canned meats, canned vegetables and Chinese style foods. While not everyone is sensitive to the effects of MSG, your health would most likely benefit from an avoidance of foods that are tainted with this additive.

While not a food itself, BPA is a toxin that comes into contact with our food and drinks via plastic dishes and storage containers. It is a chemical used in the manufacture of epoxy resins and polycarbonate plastics. Many food and liquid storage containers, such as plastic cups, baby bottles and plastic soup storage bowls, are made of plastics which contain BPA. Epoxy resins are used to line and seal the insides of vegetable and soup cans, as well as coating the supply lines that bring water into our homes. Other items that are tainted with BPA toxins include dental sealants, bottle tops and cash register receipts.

BPA seeps into food and drinks from BPA-tainted storage containers and water supply lines. Most people in industrialized nations consume or come into contact with low levels of BPA on a daily basis.

The Department of Health and Human Services' Toxicology Department has conducted research concerning the possible effects of BPA poisoning on unborn babies, infants, children and the human brain. The effects of BPA contamination are so serious that The Food and Drug Administration has stepped in and is working to reduce the amounts of BPA to which humans are exposed.

Due to the potentially damaging effects of BPA exposure, it would be wise to limit the amount of the toxin with which you come into contact. Start by eliminating BPA-containing products from your home. This may seem like a daunting task, but your efforts will be rewarded when you begin to notice your health improving.

If removing BPA products from your home is not an option for you, be sure to handle the products in the safest way possible. Do not microwave BPA plastics. (These often have the No. 7 on the bottoms of the containers.) Microwaving gradually causes the plastics to break down, which in turn causes more leeching of BPA.

BPA-containing products should be hand-washed with a mild detergent. The harsh detergents used in dishwashers have a tendency to wear down plastic containers much more quickly than hand-washing. Any type of handling that wears down the plastic may cause the BPA toxins to leech out more freely.

When possible, use stainless steel and glass containers for food storage purposes. These types of containers do not contain BPA toxins and are safe for use with foods and beverages.

Water is the fountain of life, but what happens when our drinking water is contaminated? Chlorine, fluoride and aluminum are added to water systems to help purify the water. However, these have negative side-effects. Chlorine is added to water to destroy microorganisms. Killing certain microorganisms makes drinking water healthier, but the chlorine also combines with naturally occurring materials in the water to create trihalomethanes, a substance which may trigger the development of bladder cancer. Trihalomethanes have also been linked to miscarriages in pregnant women who consumed chlorinated drinking water, as well as spina bifida and other birth defects.

Trihalomethanes can enter the human body even if the water is not consumed in the form of drinking water. When showering in chlorinated water, trihalomethanes enter the respiratory system as the evaporated water enters the air. Spending ten minutes in a hot shower can be even more dangerous than drinking a half gallon of chlorinated tap water. Showering in chlorinated water also dries out skin and contributes to hair breakage. The best way to avoid these potential problems is to use a shower filter, which will remove most of the chlorine from the water.

Fluoride is added to public drinking water to help keep tooth decay at bay, but it is also a known toxin. That is why toothpaste comes with warnings to call a poison control hotline if your child swallows too much toothpaste while brushing her teeth. Fluoride is poisonous to humans!

Aluminum is another substance used in the treatment of drinking water. It causes organic materials to clump together and makes them easier to remove from the water system. The problem with this method of cleaning water is that not all of the aluminum can be removed from the water. Therefore, aluminum remains in the water that we drink. Aluminum is harder on the human body than fluoride or chlorine. It has actually been linked to the development of Alzheimer's disease.

The question is why would our government, which is responsible for the well-being of the American people, allow, and even encourage, the use of toxins in our foods and drinking water? Is there a motive? Is there a reason our government would want us to be sick? The foods and water we consume are slowly killing us and our government agency (Food and Drug Administration) approves of it.

The only thing the people of the American public can do is take matters into our own hands and take responsibility for our health. If we continue to consume these toxins, our health will continue to decline, cancer rates will continue to climb and we will die at younger ages. There is no alternative, but to take responsibility for our own health and make the decision to no longer allow ourselves to be slowly poisoned to death.

Chapter 3- How to Improve Your Digestion

Digestive discomfort is one of the most frequent health complaints, and it can come in many forms: stomach pain, bloating, indigestion, constipation, diarrhea, and foul smelling gas. With a little understanding of how to obtain digestive health, we can eliminate most of these complaints.

Types of Fiber

Most people are not getting enough fiber in their diet; this is a shame because fiber is the single most vital nutrient needed for good digestive health. There are actually 3 different types of fiber, each with different effects on your digestive system.

Improving your digestive health is not simply a case of getting more fiber in your diet; instead, aim for a varied range of each of the three types of fiber outlined below.

Soluble fiber: This refers to fiber that dissolves in water (at least partially) to create a jelly-type substance. Soluble fiber boosts your body's ability to absorb nutrients from food by slowing down the amount of time it takes food to pass through your system. You can find soluble fiber in many kinds of fruits and vegetables (especially those with skins), as well as oats and pulses.

Insoluble fiber: Instead of dissolving in water, insoluble fiber absorbs water and does not break down. This forms the bulk of stool and helps your bowel to get rid of toxins. You can find insoluble fiber in any whole-grains foods, such as cereals and bread, as well as some kinds of fruit and vegetables.

Resistant starch: This is really important for the functioning of your intestines and bowels. It is classified as a fiber instead of a starch because it goes all the way through your intestines without breaking down. Resistant starch is good for stabilizing your blood sugar levels. You can find it in beans, firm bananas, potatoes, and pasta.

You need to ensure that you get enough fiber in your daily diet (at least 24 grams per day), but there are no specific guidelines regarding how much of each type of fiber you should ingest. Do not ban carbohydrates from your diet as this restricts you from enjoying many whole-grain and whole-wheat foods.

Good Bacteria

Our body consists of trillions and trillions of cells and yet, this is nothing compared to how much bacteria is present in our body. Some of this bacterium is bad, and some is good. Having the right balance between good and bad bacteria is vital for maintaining a healthy digestive system.

Our bodies need good bacteria (also known as probiotics) to break down the fiber in our bowels, and prompt our bowel cells to absorb essential nutrients from food.

Probiotics also promote the correct pH balance in our bodies; that is, the correct levels of acidity and alkalinity. This is crucial because our bodies function optimally when this balance is correct.

A high fiber diet encourages the growth of good bacteria in our bodies, but we can also get good bacteria directly from certain foods such as yoghurt and milk, as well as probiotic drinks and supplements.

Water

Fluids are really important in maintaining digestive health. The digestive system uses up to 10 liters of fluid; most of this is secreted from the body, but some also comes from the food and drink we consume. The majority of this fluid is reabsorbed into our bodies.

To maintain healthy digestive functioning, we need to drink between 6 and 8 glasses of water a day. You will know that you are getting enough water if your urine is pale and odorless. As insoluble fiber absorbs water, be aware that as you increase your fiber intake, you must also increase your water intake.

Pure, still water is optimal, but all hot and cold drinks can contribute as long as they do not make up the bulk of your water consumption. The exception is fruit and herbal teas; these are made entirely with hot water and are not compromised by sugar and milk.

Lifestyle

Finally, our lifestyle and general habits can affect our digestion in ways we may not even realize. For example, caffeine has a stimulating effect on our mind and body. In terms of digestion, this means that caffeine increases the speed in which foods goes through our system so that our body does not get a chance to absorb the essential nutrients from food before it enters the bowels.

Alcohol irritates your gut and upsets your bowels, whilst smoking causes muscle contractions in your bowels, which can result in diarrhea. Foods that are high in fat can cause a host of irritations, such as bloating and constipation.

In summary, the most important thing to bear in mind when considering the functioning of your digestive system is balance. We need a balance of the three primary kinds of fiber, we need a balance of good and bad bacteria, and we need our water intake to be sufficiently balanced against our fiber intake. With everything in balance, we are giving our digestive system a much needed boost, which will eliminate most of the negative effects of poor digestion.

Chapter 4- Cleaning Our Kidneys with the Right Foods – Detox Foods

Our kidneys have an incredibly important job within the body, and are in charge of cleansing our entire system of chemicals, salt, refined sugars, and even help to control our blood pressure. Often overlooked, these powerful little organs can filter up to 180 litres of blood in a single day, and do so continuously. It is up to us to ensure that they continue to function effectively, so a cleansing kidney detox is essential to our overall health. These 3 simple detox plans will cleanse the kidneys of sludge build-up, and help to treat and prevent formation of kidney stones.

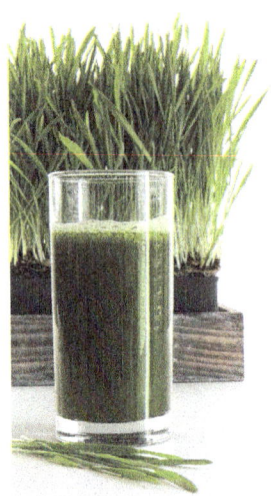

Parsley Detox

Fortunately one of the most effective methods is also the cheapest, and has many benefits besides detoxing the kidneys. Wash a bunch of fresh parsley, and then chop it into small pieces. Add the parsley to a pot of boiling water, and boil for 10 minutes. Allow the mixture to cool, and then remove the parsley using a sieve. Pour the remaining juice into a bottle or container. Refrigerate the juice, and drink one glass daily to rid the kidneys of salt and toxins. You will start to see sediment leaving the body during urination, and you will immediately begin to feel lighter, energized, and notice healthier, more radiant skin.

Dandelion Tea Detox

Dandelion has been used for centuries to treat a whole host of illnesses, yet some still regard this wonderful plant as a common weed. It is possible to buy dandelion supplements from health food shops, but as with most herbal remedies, the original plant is usually the most effective. Used throughout the world as an effective, natural way of purifying the blood, it can also be used to treat respiratory illness, arthritis, and even cancer.

If you are lucky enough to have dandelion growing close to your home, start by picking young dandelion leaves until you have enough to fill half a saucepan. Wash the leaves thoroughly, fill the saucepan with boiling water, and boil rapidly for 10 minutes. Remove the leaves, and set aside to use later in cooking or salads. Pour the tea into a container, and sweeten with honey or Stevia. The tea can be drunk hot or cold, but be sure to check with your doctor before starting this detox if you are diabetic.

Fruit Juice Detox

There are many fruit juices which are helpful in aiding kidney detox, but one of the most well-known is cranberry juice. Cranberries have natural antiseptic properties, and prevent infections from forming in the urinary tract. Make fresh cranberry juice at home using fresh or frozen cranberries. Place the washed berries in a saucepan with 1 liter of water, a few orange and lemon slices, and a pinch of salt. Boil the mixture until all of the berries have popped, then remove the fruit using a sieve and add sugar to taste. Store the mixture in the fridge and consume as often as desired. Lemons also make effective kidney cleansers, and freshly squeezed lemon juice can be added to drinking water to boost its detoxifying effects.

All of the different detox methods have at their core the same ingredient, which is pure and simple water. Doctors recommend that we drink between 8 and 10 glasses of water a day, and it is one of the main building blocks of life. It is also important to drink plenty of water whilst embarking upon a detox plan, as many have diuretic properties and can leave the body dehydrated.

Kidney disease has reached epidemic proportions over the last few decades, and our diet and lifestyle are the main culprits. A cleansing kidney detox, along with increased fresh fruit and vegetable intake, will ensure that your body remains functioning efficiently, and will set the foundations for your overall health in later life.

Chapter 5 - Understanding How to Use Free Radicals for Healthy Eating Habits

If you have ever heard of free radicals, then you probably know that they aren't good things and we should protect ourselves from them. But very few people understand the ins and outs of exactly what they are and how they can harm us. Read on for a straightforward introduction to these damaging substances.

Simply put, free radicals are abnormal oxygen molecules. They are abnormal because they have only one electron compared to the standard two. An electron is the bonding element that binds atoms together to create molecules. In simple terms, molecules are only considered to be complete and stable when its electrons are paired up. And most of the time, they are. However, sometimes bonds become weak and split in an abnormal way, thus creating an unstable molecule called a free radical.

Free radicals desperately try to become stable by attempting to attach themselves to other molecules in order to find the much needed electron. Free radicals are very quick, as they are motivated by nothing other than maximizing their stability by finding a second electron (even if this means stealing an electron from another molecule). They will always attack the first molecule they come across. If this molecule is unprotected, it will lose one of its electrons and become a free radical itself. This process can continue in a chain reaction, or domino effect. This can become a serious problem if the first molecule a free radical comes across happens to be an important one such as DNA molecules.

Free radicals are a normal part of life and they are present in the environment. Free radicals enter our bodies on a daily basis, from cigarette smoke, pollution, germs, certain foods and drinks etc. The human body is normally able to deal with moderate levels of free radicals. However, if free radical damage becomes severe, we can become susceptible to many kinds of diseases.

The Role of Antioxidants

The fight against free radicals is not a lost cause. Antioxidants are molecules that protect our bodies from free radical damage by putting a stop to the chain reaction of electron stealing that free radicals cause. They do this by giving up one of their own electrons to the free radical, effectively rendering it neutralized, stabilized and harmless. After interaction with an antioxidant, a free radical will no longer try to steal electrons from the healthy cells in our body because the antioxidant has willingly given it what it was looking for.

So now that we have established the role of antioxidants in protecting us against the negative effects of free radicals, the next logical question to answer is "where can we find antioxidants?" Well, the simplest and most effective way to incorporate antioxidants into your system is by eating foods that are rich in these special nutrients and contain almost no free radicals at all. Typically these include fruit and vegetables, as well as nuts and seeds. Brightly colored foods such as tomatoes and greens are considered to be the most concentrated examples of antioxidants. Antioxidants include a whole variety of vitamins and minerals and it is important to vary the colors of foods you eat to get a well-rounded supply.

So we've discovered that free radicals are actually molecules that have only one electron, compared to the usual two electrons. To compensate for this, free radicals search for a health cell in which they can steal an electron. In modest doses, our bodies can keep free radicals under control, especially if our diet is rich in antioxidants which willingly give up one of their electrons to the scavenging free radical. The bottom line seems to be that the more healthy foods we eat, the greater our antioxidant intake will be, which in turn will determine how effectively our bodies fight against the damaging effects of free radicals.

Chapter 6- The Truth about Healthy Cholesterols

Heart attacks and strokes affect the lives of millions of people, and many of them thought they were living healthy lives before illness struck. A common belief is that if cholesterol levels are within normal range, the risk of serious illness is low. In reality, having normal or low levels of cholesterol does not eliminate the risk of a heart attack or stroke.

Many of the myths about cholesterol levels are created by the drugs industry. Cholesterol lowering drugs are a multi-billion dollar industry, and the companies profiting are keen to promote the belief that they can prevent serious illness. In reality, cholesterol is a vital component in the body, and is needed to keep you alive.

The key to a healthy heart is getting the balance of the 'good' and 'bad' types of cholesterol in your body. Cholesterol has many important functions within the body, including helping nerves to function correctly and maintaining strong cell membranes. Mainstream medicine's solution to reducing cholesterol levels is generally drugs which block the production of cholesterol in your liver. As well as having worrying side effects, there is a danger these drugs can take cholesterol levels too low.

When cholesterol levels are too low, there are risks of memory loss, dementia and depression. In some studies, there is evidence of increased risks of behavioral changes, unbalanced hormone levels and even cancer.

With all of this confusing information, how can we actually maintain healthy cholesterol levels? Cholesterol doesn't dissolve directly in blood, and is carried around the body in little packages. These biological packages are called lipoproteins, and understanding the two types is crucial to understanding healthy cholesterol levels. Low density lipoproteins (LDL) are the 'bad' type, and high density lipoproteins (HDL) are the 'good' ones. The key is simply to keep LDL at low levels and HDL at high levels.

Maintaining a healthy balance between HDL and LDL is very much in line with what most people believe to be living a healthy lifestyle. Taking regular exercise is a good way to start. Walking, swimming, weight-lifting and general aerobic exercise are great steps forward in improving cholesterol levels. Stopping smoking, lowering alcohol intake and reducing stress are further ways you can begin the journey to healthy cholesterol balance.

Nutrients and vitamins are the perfect alternative to man-made drugs for tackling cholesterol problems. Small changes in diet can make a big difference. A diet low in saturated fats and carbohydrates is the long-term solution, and can reduce many other health risks at the same time. Contrary to what many people believe, avoiding high-cholesterol foods doesn't immediately lower cholesterol levels. A mechanism in the human body regulates production of cholesterol, and less is produced when more is eaten. High carbohydrate diets rich in white bread and pasta are a greater danger than eating eggs and meat as some people believe.

Eating oily fish such as salmon and mackerel is another great way to tackle cholesterol concerns. These can be taken in supplement form if you don't like eating fish. Foods rich in fiber, soya, garlic and niacin also have proven benefits in controlling cholesterol levels.

Chapter 7- Top Ten Tips for a Healthier You

When it comes to being healthier, there is no time like the present. You won't become the face of perfect health overnight, so why try to reinvent your life in a day? You won't find radical changes in this article and you won't be nagged to quit long term habits or to make life changing sacrifices. The tips presented in this article are very simple things you can do today to boost your physical health a little bit at a time. Incorporate these small but significant changes into your life will dramatically improve your health.

Reduce the amount of sugar you add to your tea or coffee. A balanced diet means everything in moderation. Ask yourself how many hot beverages you drink on a typical day and how many spoons of sugar you add to each drink. An average person could be putting 6-10 spoons of sugar into their body every day. So if you usually add two spoons of sugar, do yourself a favor today and half that to one.

Pour yourself a glass of water. Adequate hydration is the most important step to becoming healthier. Every single function of every single organ in your body relies on water. Therefore the most beneficial thing you can do today is to drink a little more water. Your body will absolutely thank you for it.

Many modern families eat their dinner in front of the TV. With your attention split between watching TV and eating, you are less able to control the speed with which you eat. As a result, you may rush and end up feeling bloated. Instead, sit at the table and focus on enjoying the taste of your meal. This will encourage you to eat your food slower and chew more thoroughly. In turn, your digestion will be greatly improved because it benefits from foods that have been completely broken down into soft, manageable chunks.

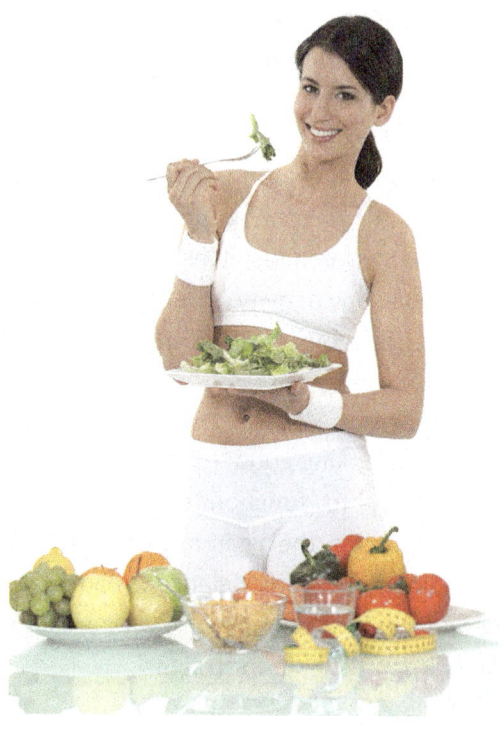

Don't skip breakfast. With the usual morning rush, many people don't have time for breakfast and just grab a cappuccino on their way to work. Caffeine can certainly help to stay alert and awake during the day. Fortunately, having breakfast can do this task equally well, if not better. Aim to eat breakfast within 2 hours of waking for maximum benefit. Eating breakfast kick starts your metabolism, meaning that you will burn off calories faster. If you choose a low sugar, high fiber breakfast, you can enjoy greater and more sustainable energy throughout the day.

Eat a piece of fruit and add some vegetables to your dinner. Getting your 5 a day isn't always easy, but we can at least try to get a few portions into our diet. Even an apple after lunch and some frozen peas with dinner will be far better than nothing.

Learning to breathe properly will boost your energy levels, calm your mind and assist your immune system. You don't need to buy anything and you don't even need to leave your desk. Focus on breathing deeply and evenly, trying to match the length of the exhales to the length of the inhales.

A general guideline is that we should exercise for at least 30 minutes every day for optimal health. The last time you exercised is irrelevant. It doesn't matter what has gone before. There is no time like the present to change. It doesn't have to be a complicated series of cardio workouts; any activity is better than nothing. So go for a walk or a jog, dance around your living room, or play in the garden with your kids.

Posture is not just about looking good; it is very important in terms of promoting your body to function correctly. Good posture involves correctly positioning the ligaments and muscles in your back so that your spine is properly balanced. Bad posture causes your spine to put unnecessary pressure on your nervous system. To avoid a trip to the chiropractor, sit up straight!

If you spend most of you time indoors, go outside for 10 minutes today and breathe in the fresh air. This will promote healthy functioning of the lungs because fresh air encourages your lungs to dilate more fully, which allows more oxygen to enter. In turn, your energy levels will naturally increase.

Stretching your muscles is fantastic for your physical health and fitness. The loosening of muscles prepares them for activity and prevents injuries from occurring during exercise. If you often experience soreness and tension in your muscles after exercises, you will find that regular stretching for 5-10 minutes each day will help to eliminate these pains.

Arguably, these 10 suggestions for improving your physical health are not hugely inconvenient or overwhelming additions to your life.

Jason Craig

In fact, they are quite minor changes which produce comparatively large benefits. Do yourself a world of good and ensure that you practice at least a few of these healthy habits every day.

About The Author

Jason Craig grew up eating lots of unhealthy foods and as such he had to struggle with his weight. He remembered being extremely frustrated and went through numerous diets trying to lose the unwanted fat.

From all of his efforts he soon realized that the solution was in what he was consuming and the amount of exercise that he was getting. Bad foods would hurt the system and good foods would help heal. All that he had to do was to modify the diet to more healthy options and the solution was as simple as that.

Jason was eager to share the success that he had had with this process and believes that it can work for any individual as long as they are dedicated to the process. He reminds the reader that things do not happen in day and that it will take time to get the body back to a healthy balance.